<u>Navigating the Challenges of Long COVID: Understanding its Causes and Impact</u>

Hey there, folks! Today, let's dive into a topic that's been on everyone's minds lately: Long COVID.

You've probably heard about it in the news or maybe even know someone who's been affected by it.

But what exactly is it, and why does it happen? And perhaps more importantly, how does it affect us humans? Let's break it down in a conversational manner.

<u>What is Long COVID, Anyway?</u>

So, you know how COVID-19 is caused by the pesky little virus called SARS-CoV-2? Well, Long COVID, or post-acute sequelae of SARS-CoV-2 infection (PASC), is what happens when the symptoms of COVID-19 stick around long after the initial infection has cleared up.

It's like the virus decides to overstay its welcome in our bodies, leaving us dealing with a whole bunch of not-so-fun symptoms.

How Does Long COVID Happen?

Now, let's get into the nitty-gritty of how this whole long COVID thing happens.

 There are a few theories floating around, but here are the main ones:

Immune System Gone Haywire:

So, our immune system is pretty awesome at fighting off infections, right? But sometimes, it can get a bit too excited and go into overdrive.

In the case of COVID-19, some folks' immune systems just can't seem to chill out even after the virus is gone.

This leads to chronic inflammation, which can cause all sorts of issues and keep those symptoms lingering.

Virus Playing Hide and Seek:

Another possibility is that the virus itself is playing tricks on us.

It might be hiding out in certain nooks and crannies of our bodies, like the respiratory or nervous systems, where our immune system can't quite reach it.

This sneaky behavior can lead to ongoing tissue damage and inflammation, keeping the symptoms going strong.

Blood Vessel Blues:

 COVID-19 has a knack for messing with our blood vessels, causing endothelial dysfunction.

 This basically means our blood vessels aren't working as they should, which can lead to all sorts of problems like impaired circulation and tissue damage.

 And you guessed it, these issues can contribute to the development of long-term symptoms.

How Does Long COVID Affect Us Humans?

Now, let's talk about the real deal: how long COVID affects us humans.

It's not just about feeling a bit under the weather for a few extra days.

Nope, it can have some pretty serious impacts on our lives. Here are a few ways it can shake things up:

Feeling Tired All The Time:

Imagine waking up every day feeling like you've been hit by a truck.

That's what some folks with long COVID experience. Fatigue so intense it feels like your body just can't keep up.

And it's not just a little tiredness – it's a bone-deep exhaustion that makes even the simplest tasks feel like climbing Mount Everest.

Brain Fog Central:

 Ever had one of those days where you can't seem to string a coherent thought together?

 Well, imagine feeling like that all the time.

 Brain fog is a common symptom of long COVID, leaving folks struggling with memory problems, difficulty concentrating, and just feeling downright foggy-headed.

Breathing Battles:

 Shortness of breath and chest tightness aren't just reserved for the acute phase of COVID-19.

 Nope, they can stick around long after the virus is gone, making it feel like you're constantly gasping for air.

 It's not exactly a walk in the park when even the simplest tasks leave you feeling winded.

Mental Health Rollercoaster:

 Dealing with a chronic illness like long COVID can take a serious toll on your mental health.

 Anxiety, depression, and stress are common companions for folks navigating the ups and downs of this condition.

 It's not just about the physical symptoms – it's about the emotional toll it takes on you as well.

Tip of The Tongue Syndrome:

 Let's talk about something that's been dubbed the "tip of the tongue syndrome" of long COVID.

 You know that frustrating feeling when you just can't quite remember a word, even though it's right there on the tip of your tongue?

 Well, imagine that feeling, but instead of lasting for a few seconds, it sticks around for weeks or even months.

So, what exactly is this "tip of the tongue syndrome" in the context of long COVID?

Well, it's one of those sneaky symptoms that can linger long after the acute phase of the illness has passed.

People with long COVID often report experiencing cognitive symptoms like brain fog and memory problems as mentioned, and this tip-of-the-tongue phenomenon is just one example.

Imagine trying to have a conversation or write an email, and you keep getting stuck on words that should be right at your fingertips.

It's like your brain is playing a game of hide and seek with your vocabulary, and sometimes, it feels like the words are just out of reach.

This symptom can be incredibly frustrating and even embarrassing at times.

You know the word you want to say, but it's like there's a mental block preventing you from retrieving it.

It can make communication feel like an uphill battle, leaving you feeling frustrated and defeated.

But here's the thing: you're not alone. Many people with long COVID experience this tip-of-the-tongue phenomenon, along with a whole host of other cognitive symptoms.

And while it can be challenging to deal with, it's important to remember that it's just another part of the journey toward recovery.

<u>Wrapping It Up</u>

So, there you have it, folks. Long COVID may be a relatively new phenomenon, but it's already making waves in the world of healthcare.

 Understanding how it happens and its impact on us humans is crucial for providing support and finding ways to manage the symptoms.

 It's a tough road to navigate, but with a little understanding and a whole lot of support, we'll get through it together.

Please use the next few pages for your notes and debates.